How I lost 155 Pounds in 10 Months

A life overshadowed by weight

Brian Encarnacion

Contents

Disclaimer

This book shares the author's personal weight loss journey and is not intended as professional health or medical advice. Readers should consult healthcare professionals before making any lifestyle changes. The author and publisher are not liable for any outcomes from using the information in this book.

Prologue

A Life Overshadowed by Weight

My name is Brian; I want to share the story of my rigorous battle with obesity, a struggle that significantly overshadowed every aspect of my life. From my earliest memories, my family's possibly unintentional ridicule planted seeds of shame and insecurity within me. Their supposedly light-hearted jokes heavily burdened my young heart, ultimately embedding a deep sense of worthlessness in my soul.

As I stepped out into the wider world, my challenges grew. In elementary school, I faced relentless bullying. A particularly vivid and painful memory was discovering a large pig nose someone had drawn on my desk. Walking into the classroom to the sound of classmates oinking was traumatic, making me feel utterly alone and vulnerable. The person responsible never came forward, and the laughter in the hallways seemed to mock my helplessness.

In high school, cruel and hurtful name-calling ensued, leaving deep scars on my psyche. Proms, parties, and events others enjoyed were alien to me. My exclusion from these functions constantly reminded me of my isolation. College offered no relief. There, among a sea of faces, I remained the invisible one, always overlooked and never chosen. Being the last one to be picked for group projects and studies underscored my evident loneliness, reinforcing my self-imposed exile.

After graduating at twenty-five, I entered the professional world, working at a business process outsourcing company. But even this new chapter did not spare me from feelings of exclusion. I found refuge in video games, a world away from judgmental stares and whispers.

At twenty-seven, I weighed 320 pounds at a height of 5 foot 10 inches. Each pound was a stark reminder of years of self-neglect. My social life was non-existent, leaving me feeling like an outsider, looking into a world where I didn't belong. My relationship with food was complex, a mix of emotional reliance and poor choices. Despite trying numerous diets and fitness trends, I never achieved much-needed lasting results. I would start a new diet and exercise regime, even buying meal supplements and equipment, but I always found myself quitting by day two. My diet mainly consisted of fast food and solitary, hurried meals in my car or room, hidden from prying eyes.

Shopping for clothes was an ongoing struggle, filled with embarrassment as I searched for hard-to-find sizes, reminding me of my failures.

Despite doctors' urgent warnings about my borderline hypertension and high sugar levels, I remained in denial, ignoring the apparent harm I was doing to my body. In this life, burdened by physical and emotional weight, the idea of change seemed impossible. Yet, I was about to realize that even the deepest habits and beliefs can be challenged and changed. This story isn't just about weight loss; it's a journey of facing and overcoming my greatest adversary—myself.

CHAPTER 1

The Catalyst of Friendship and Heartache

My life was nothing extraordinary other than my size, driving to and from work every day, Mondays to Fridays. Confined to the 4 corners of my cubicle, answering phone calls. Going on breaks, frequenting the pantry and cafeteria nearby. My pedestal was filled with goods and treats, almost like a mini pantry on its own.

My station was positioned along the hallway where co-workers passed by frequently, but oddly, I can't remember any of them saying a Hi or Hello without feeling awkward when my eyes caught their attention.

At home after work, I'd be locking myself in my room, playing my video games with pizza next to me and a 6 pack can of soda. That was life to me back then—the same thing day in and day out.

Everything began to change the day Mark, a new co-worker, offered me genuine friendship. Free from the usual pity or disdain I had grown accustomed to, his approach radiated warmth and sincerity. This simple act of kindness shone brightly in my otherwise dim and lonely world.

One day, a tall, slender, and fair-skinned guy with full black hair and very Asian type of eyes - Mark, approached my cubicle and invited me to lunch with a friendly smile, saying, "Hey, Brian, join me for lunch. Will you? I could really enjoy some good company." His eyes sparkled with a sincerity that felt both new and comforting. This invitation was unlike any I had ever received before. I hesitated, my heart racing with a mixture of hope and apprehension. Past betrayals, where people approached me with hidden motives, clouded my judgment. Was this genuine? "Are you sure? I mean, yeah, I'd love to join you. Thanks, Mark. That means a lot," I replied, my voice a mixture of surprise and cautious optimism. Though seemingly minor, this interaction felt like a pivotal moment in my life

—a door opening to possibilities and friendships I had never dared to hope for.

In the past, there've been several encounters where people befriended me with hidden motives, and I often end up heartbroken, either romantically or just as friends. I remember this one guy I thought I was dating in my neighborhood, tall and handsome, befriending me and making me feel important. I almost completely fell for him. After gaining my trust, he borrowed a huge amount of money but never returned it or showed up. Not answering my calls, messages, or texts, ignoring me, and passing me by. I never got the courage to talk to him as I felt ashamed and utterly stupid.

As Mark and I began spending more time together, I discovered a friendship based on genuine connection and mutual respect. He looked past my physical appearance and connected with me on a deeper level. We quickly found common ground in our love for video games, anime, and music, forming the foundation of our growing friendship. We spent many lunch breaks and after-work hours engaged in passionate discussions about our favorite games and anime series, moments I eagerly anticipated.

Mark's tales of his romantic escapades and vibrant social life opened a window to a world both exciting and foreign to me. Captivated, I listened as he described his adventures, the parties he attended, and the people he met. These stories ignited a desire in me to know more about him and, more importantly, to start seeking similar experiences for myself.

Mark's influence went beyond our one-on-one interactions. He gradually introduced me to other colleagues, helping me become part of a diverse, helpful, and welcoming group at work. Their acceptance and warmth gradually unraveled the layers of isolation I had wrapped around myself over the years. Joining in on daily conversations, laughing together at jokes, and simply being part of a group made me feel more visible and valued than ever before. For the first time in a long time, I didn't feel like an outsider looking in; I felt like I belonged.

However, as weeks turned into months, my feelings for Mark evolved into something deeper. I began developing romantic feelings for him, a blend of exhilaration and fear I had never fully experienced. I wrestled with these feelings, uncertain of their reciprocation but unable to suppress them.

After much internal debate, I decided to share my feelings with Mark. "Mark, there's something important I need to tell you," I said one day, my heart pounding with fear and hope. We found a quiet corner, and I gathered my courage. "Mark, you've become an incredibly important person in my life. You see me for who I am, not just my appearance. Over time, I've started to feel something more for you, something deeper than I've ever felt for anyone else," I confessed, my voice trembling with vulnerability.

Mark listened with empathy, his face showing compassion and surprise. After a thoughtful pause, he responded with gentleness and honesty. "Brian, I'm deeply touched by your words. You're an amazing person, and I value our friendship immensely. But I don't share those romantic feelings. I truly hope this doesn't affect our great friendship," he said sincerely.

In that moment, I felt an overwhelming sense of rejection. It felt like all the years of pain, ridicule, and loneliness had come crashing down on me. The sincerity in Mark's words was overshadowed by a mountain of haunting memories—the years of being bullied, feeling invisible, and overlooked. The sting of unrequited love was not just about the present moment; it was a painful reminder of all the past hurts I had never fully overcome. This realization was devastating, igniting a fierce determination within me. I was angry, not just at the situation but at all the years of accumulated pain and hurt.

This anger transformed into a powerful catalyst. It immensely propelled me to make a life-altering decision: to transform myself, not for someone else but for my own well- being and happiness. I set a bold and ambitious goal for myself: to lose weight and take control of my life once and for all.

CHAPTER 2
The Gym

Destiny seemed to nudge me forward when a high-end gym opened just a few minutes' walk from my office. Its sleek design and welcoming atmosphere stood out as a beacon of hope, offering a path away from the shadows of unrequited love and the enduring scars of schoolyard bullying that had clung to me for years.

With anticipation and intense nervousness, I stepped into what would become my sanctuary for transformation. Entering the gym and signing up, I felt overwhelmed with emotions. The staff greeted me warmly! Their cheerfulness made it feel like a reunion with a long-lost friend. Joining this gym wasn't just signing up for exercise; it was a commitment to a new beginning, a pledge to heal from the wounds of unreciprocated love and past bullying.

The very next day, I found myself at the back of an exercise studio, clad in oversized workout gear, ready for my first group exercise class—Mixed Martial Arts - an intense 1- hour cardio workout that lets you punch and kick your way toward your fitness goals. To bolster my wavering confidence, I whispered to myself, "You can do this! It's easy!" Despite my nervousness, my determination to reinvent myself and shed the layers of my past life was clear.

Reality struck hard and fast. Within minutes of the class starting, I was gasping for breath, drenched in sweat, and my heart was racing profusely. The class's intensity shocked my system. What I intended to be a short break turned into a twenty-minute retreat to catch my breath. Rejoining the class, I soon found myself needing another pause. It was a physical challenge, unlike anything I had ever faced.

As I returned home that evening, I felt the familiar urge to reward myself with food. Convincing myself I had earned it, I indulged in a massive pizza and soda, rationalizing it as a well-deserved treat for my hard work, rewarding myself with food after a workout session sabotaging my fitness efforts.

Feeling sore and justifying a break the next day, I skipped the gym. This pattern continued, and before I knew it, a whole week had passed without me returning. That first Mixed Martial Arts class ended up being my last.

I felt like I had slipped back into my old habits. Sitting in front of my computer at the office, a quiet voice inside me urged, "Go back to the gym." Glancing at my workout bag, packed and ready since last week, I couldn't find the motivation to pick it up. Then, Mark passed by, casually asking, "Hey, how's it going?"

Suddenly, a flood of emotions washed over me—memories of bullying, being ridiculed about my size, and all the times I had started and failed to change. These realizations and mixed emotions pushed me to return to the gym. In the locker room, I questioned myself, "What just happened? I saw Mark, and suddenly, I felt the urge to come here?" It struck me that relying on sporadic encounters with Mark for motivation wasn't sustainable. I needed to make gym attendance a regular part of my life.

Feeling intimidated in the gym, surrounded by experienced gym-goers, I wanted to escape. Their grunts and shouts made them seem like titans. But then, thinking of Mark and my new friends, I realized that intimidation shouldn't hold me back. I reminded myself, "Everyone here started where I am now. If I don't get going today, I'll never reach their level, and that's where I want to be."

Embracing my inner nerd, I indulged in my love for data analysis and tracking. Using these skills, I created a detailed spreadsheet accessible on my laptop and phone to track my gym habits. This wasn't just about my performance in the gym; it was about showing up consistently. True to my analytical nature, I took joy in filling out this tracker after each gym session. Initially aiming for three times a week, my gym attendance soon evolved into a daily routine.

A month later, with consistent tracking and gym visits, I found myself stronger, lasting longer in classes, and climbing stairs with ease. I realized that while strong motivation can kickstart a journey, it's building a solid habit that keeps you going.

Understanding the science of resistance training boosted my experience. Just as muscles grow stronger, more robust, and more resilient through regular workouts, forming a habit requires consistent effort and dedication. Each gym session was like a rep in a workout, strengthening not just my body but my resolve and discipline. This habit- building process mirrored the principles of progressive overload in resistance training— gradual increases in stress on the body lead to increased strength and endurance over time. By applying this concept to my gym routine, I was not only building physical strength but also resilience in maintaining my new lifestyle.

Feeling empowered and stronger than ever, I eagerly anticipated my next weigh-in, ready to face the scale after a month of newfound discipline and determination.

Chapter 3

Diet Overhaul!

When I first opened my eyes to the world, my father had already retired from twenty years of valiant service in the Navy. In this new chapter of his life, he donned the chef's hat, infusing our home with his passion for cooking. He shared not just his time with me but also his culinary expertise, a legacy I hold dear.

I vividly remember him returning from the US Commissary, laden with American groceries that couldn't be found in our local Philippine markets. The variety of sweet treats and chocolates he brought home were not mere food items; they symbolized a privileged childhood, rare delights most kids in our neighborhood could only dream of.

Each year, on their wedding anniversary, my father would lovingly prepare six chickens, one for each of us siblings, irrespective of our age, size, or appetite. This tradition exemplified our family's abundance, a tangible expression of our parents' love. They were determined to spare us the deprivation they had known in their own childhood.

As a child, food meant more than nourishment to me; it was an affirmation of true love. Every bite I savored, every additional serving I requested, seemed to reinforce the bond of love between my parents and me.

As I grew older, food became a source of comfort. Whether returning from school weary or from work draped in melancholy, my parents were always there, offering solace in the form of succulent rib-eye steaks with fluffy mashed potatoes, and indulgent desserts. This ritual of eating in response to fatigue, sadness, or the agony of being bullied at school became my main source of relief.

As my parents aged and cooked less frequently, I found myself uncontrollably turning to these familiar comfort foods all the more. I bought them, prepared them, and consumed them. The habit of eating when stressed, sad, or depressed had taken root deep within me. "Eating your emotions away" perfectly encapsulated my coping mechanism.

Realizing that this habit was deep-rooted and stemmed from childhood adversities marked a crucial turning point in my life. I came to understand that losing weight wasn't just about changing my diet; it was about recognizing the emotional underpinnings of my eating habits.

A month into my gym routine, heavy frustration started to mount. My weight stubbornly resisted change despite noticeable improvements in strength and stamina. The scale's refusal to budge led to a moment of childlike despair—I literally stomped out of the gym, feeling utterly defeated. This was the moment that drove me to seek answers, leading to a critical realization: my diet was the main barrier in my weight loss journey. The advice of a fitness consultant, which I had initially overlooked, suddenly became my guiding light.

Delving into introspection and extensive online research, I discovered the concepts of Basal Metabolic Rate (BMR) and Total Daily Energy Expenditure (TDEE). BMR, the calories burned at rest, highlighted the importance of having a clear understanding of individual caloric needs. TDEE, incorporating daily activities and lifestyle, showed how energy needs varied with physical activity levels.

For instance, someone with a BMR of 1500 calories who leads a lightly active lifestyle would have a TDEE of approximately 2062.5 calories (1500 x 1.375). This knowledge prompted me to critically analyze my daily food intake:

- Breakfast: Three pancakes, six strips of bacon, six hash browns – 1800 calories

- Lunch: Burger, pizza slice, fries, soda – 1500 calories

- Dinner: Spaghetti and meatballs, fried chicken, pie, soda – 2000 calories

This totaled over 5000 calories daily, far exceeding both my BMR and TDEE. Although this wasn't my everyday intake, it represented the typical abundance of my meals. Further research highlighted the emotional impact of consuming high-sugar and carbohydrate foods, which triggered a cycle of dopamine-induced highs and lows.

Embracing this newfound understanding, I began my diet overhaul with a symbolic meal: grilled chicken breast, steamed broccoli, and brown rice. The flavors were subtler than the fast food I was accustomed to, marking the start of a transformative chapter in my life. The first week was the most challenging, battling against my habits of comfort eating, meticulously counting calories, and measuring portions. Moments of doubt and temptation tortuously tested my resolve. I remember this one time I thought I was about to snap; I was near the drive-through of McDonald's, staring at its golden arches, contemplating what to order after a good gym session. I was heavily thinking about fries, a hot fudge sundae, and a Big Mac till I slapped myself crazy, grabbed my yogurt next to me, and drove away.

In social settings, I learned to navigate my dietary goals with support from understanding friends and family. Even Mark, who had once rejected my love confession, showed immense support. Friends chose places accommodating my dietary needs, and family gatherings gradually became supportive of my new lifestyle. Fortunately, we were able to find a cafeteria near work where they served an array of healthier options and food choices, including many different kinds of salads.

This journey transcended changing what I ate; it marked a profound transformation of my relationship with food. Armed with a deeper understanding of BMR and TDEE, along with a clear awareness of the dopamine sugar rush, I made informed, healthier choices, leading to a more balanced and fulfilling life. Whenever a strong emotional pull tempted me to revert to my old eating habits, I relied on my motivation and newfound knowledge. I constantly reminded myself of the damage I had done to my body and resolved not to repeat past mistakes. I refused to fall back into old patterns.

Though I occasionally slipped up, the decreasing numbers on the scale further motivated me. I also found a new source of fulfillment in working out and exercising, replacing the temporary comfort I once found in food.

Chapter 4

Embracing Change – The Many Types of Exercise!

As the weeks turned into months, I diversified my exercise routine. Mixing up my workouts proved crucial for maintaining both physical and mental engagement. Each form of exercise targeted different muscle groups, improved various aspects of fitness like flexibility, strength, and cardiovascular health, and reduced the risk of overuse injuries. It also kept my routine fresh and exciting, preventing boredom and burnout. Incorporating dance, yoga, and other activities into my fitness regime enhanced not only my physical capabilities but also contributed to a more holistic sense of well-being.

Having a clear understanding of the role of various workout types in the context of a comprehensive fitness plan was pivotal. Cardiovascular exercises improved my heart health and stamina, while weightlifting focused on building muscle strength and mass. Activities like yoga and Pilates offered flexibility and core strength, which are vital for overall fitness and injury prevention. Each workout type played a unique role, collectively contributing to a well-rounded fitness regime.

This variety also kept my mind engaged. The challenge of learning new skills and breaking the monotony of a single type of exercise kept me motivated. It was fascinating to see how different activities complemented each other—strength training made me more robust for my yoga sessions, while the flexibility gained from yoga improved my range of motion for weightlifting.

Eight months into this transformative journey, after overcoming numerous challenges and maintaining unwavering dedication, I reached a significant milestone. The scale now read 165 pounds, a figure that stood as a testament to the effectiveness of a balanced approach to weight loss, combining diet and exercise. This achievement reflected the incredible support system around me, the inner strength I harnessed, and my relentless commitment to a once unattainable goal.

The support of friends and family played a pivotal role in the success I achieved. My family being mindful of what they prepare for lunch, making sure that I don't get tempted by what they serve on the table, and my work friends always considering me when it comes to dining out and enjoying our time together. Both my family and friends constantly pushing me to go to the gym whenever they feel I'm slacking. Finding a community that understood and supported my goals made a significant difference. Their encouragement and willingness to adapt to my dietary needs were crucial in maintaining my motivation and commitment to my health journey.

The gym had transformed into more than just a workout space; it became a place of education and self-exploration. It was here that I began to intelligibly grasp the intricate interplay between physical activity, nutrition, and emotional well-being. This realization marked the onset of a more comprehensive approach to my weight loss journey, significantly prompting me to address and alter deep-rooted habits and beliefs.

This chapter of my journey was about more than losing weight; it was about gaining a stronger sense of self, a deeper understanding of my body, and an unshakable belief in the possibility of change. As I looked back at my progress, I realized this was just the beginning of a lifelong commitment to health, well-being, and self-discovery.

CHAPTER 5

Awakening

As the days turned into weeks and the weeks into months, my reflection in the mirror began to reveal someone I hardly recognized—someone who stood taller, smiled more, and exuded unprecedented confidence. I began to feel a sense of liberation, not just from the physical weight but from the mental chains that had bound me for so long. I was no longer the man who regularly hid behind baggy clothes, avoided eye contact, or felt unworthy of attention and love.

This self-assurance was more than skin deep. It was discovering entire parts of myself that had long been dormant. I found myself readily engaging in conversations more freely, no longer shrinking away from attention but welcoming it. The once daunting task of walking into a room full of strangers transformed into an exciting opportunity to meet new people and make connections. The changes in my physical appearance were undeniable, but the changes within me were even more profound.

My transformation journey also led me to rediscover and cultivate new interests and hobbies. Activities like walking, jogging, going to parks, and meeting people—which I had previously viewed with apprehension or indifference—now became sources of immense pleasure and pride. They were no longer just means to burn calories and move but activities that enriched my life and broadened my horizons.

A pivotal aspect of my transformation journey was the meticulous tracking of my habits. I embraced technology, such as using mobile devices and laptops to use spreadsheets and fitness apps to track my progress and monitor my diet. This practice of recording and reviewing my progress became a ritual that not only kept me accountable but also provided immense satisfaction. It was a concrete representation of my journey, an important map that showed where I had started and how far I had come.

The transformation brought about a wave of external validation and admiration, which, while uplifting, also taught me an important lesson about self-worth. It acknowledged my hard work and dedication. Sometimes, I'd pass by a building with windows and have to do a doubletake at my reflection, as I hardly recognized myself.

I was awakening to a new sense of self—a new way of existing in the world. And I loved every minute of it...

CHAPTER 6

The Price of Transformation

The progressive transformation I underwent brought an avalanche of attention and admiration I had never experienced before. At work, I suddenly found myself in the limelight, constantly receiving applause and recognition from colleagues and bosses who previously seemed to barely notice me. My family, too, joined in this chorus of praise, sometimes inadvertently overshadowing the achievements of other family members. All of this attention felt surreal, and for the first time in my life, I felt truly seen and acknowledged. I relished this newfound celebrity-like status.

With the attention came an unexpected form of admiration for my physical appearance. It was exhilarating and unfamiliar. I felt unstoppable, riding a continuous high of newfound confidence and vitality. This newfound self-assurance propelled me into the dating scene with gusto, moving from one relationship to the next, savoring the thrill and excitement of each new encounter.

Once a dreaded activity, shopping transformed into a delightful experience. I reveled in the freedom of choosing clothes from any store, selecting sizes I had never dreamed possible before. This stark contrast to the days of searching for quadruple-X sizes filled me with a sense of triumph.

Clubbing, an experience I previously thought was reserved for others, became a regular part of my weekends. I immersed myself in the vibrant nightlife, enjoying the attention and living what I once thought only happened in movies. Scenes that were once mere fantasies became my reality. Dancing in the club, catching the eye of the most attractive person there, and sharing a spontaneous kiss amidst the pulsating lights

—these were no longer just wishful thoughts.

I remember this one time I had a blind date. He was tall and almost looked like one of those super-hot Korean/Chinese actors you'd see on social media that everyone would be drooling over. When we introduced each other outside the bar, I felt he was out of my league. I immediately escaped after the pleasantries, believing he wasn't going to be interested in me. I went inside the club, by the bar, drinking my self-pity away. A few moments later, the guy I came inside, pulled me to the dance floor, danced me away, staring into my eyes, and all of a sudden kissed me. Everything turned grey, and the party music faded to a single hum. It was one of the most exhilarating feelings in my life.

However, this intoxicating influx of attention and admiration soon became addictive. I found myself craving more validation, constantly seeking approval for my physical appearance. Despite achieving my initial weight loss goal, I pushed myself further, pursuing even more weight loss.

As my weight dropped from 165 pounds to 160 pounds, concern began to surface among some friends and family members. They noted my increasingly gaunt appearance, but I dismissed their worries as envy or misunderstanding. Ten months later, I weighed 155 lbs. Now, even my closest friends and loved ones expressed alarm. I stubbornly ignored their warnings, convinced they couldn't comprehend the euphoria of my accomplishments.

Amidst the flurry of social activities and relationships, a profound sense of emptiness persisted. None of these fleeting connections filled the hollow void within me. Then, one day, in a relentless pursuit of further weight loss, I found myself in the bathroom, inducing vomiting.

After the fact, the sight of my hair falling out and the stark realization of my actions hit me with devastating force. I collapsed to the floor, engulfed in sadness, finally recognizing the extent of my obsession.

This moment of painful clarity marked a turning point. What had begun as a quest for a healthier life had dangerously veered into a terrible obsession, a fixation that was no longer about physical health but a battle with mental well-being. This realization was the first step in acknowledging that my journey had taken a perilous turn, and it was time to seek help and reclaim not just my physical health but my mental and emotional well-being as well.

CHAPTER 7

Rediscovering Self-Love

Paradoxically, reaching my goal weight, a milestone I had longed for, did not bring the fulfillment I had anticipated. Instead, I found myself engulfed in a sea of self- reflection, questioning the essence of the person I had become. The relentless chase for attention and validation had steered me off course—far from my true self. It was a startling realization that I had unwittingly placed external validation above my own health and well-being in my quest.

During this period of deep introspection, I turned to yoga, seeking a path to a more profound sense of balance and self-awareness. Guided by a compassionate teacher, my yoga journey evolved into a sanctuary of self-discovery. Yoga transcended the realm of physical exercise; it became a quest for inner tranquility and understanding. On the yoga mat, I learned the art of harmonizing body and mind, unveiling a path to authentic health that transcends physical appearance.

You see, I've been regularly doing yoga as part of my fitness regimen, but I never fully understood its deeper and more profound benefits until I genuinely listened to my teacher. In one particular class, after my meltdown, as I was doing a yoga posture that was challenging and difficult, the yoga teacher said, "As you stay into the pose, feel how challenging it is for your body. Feel how tight you are and how difficult it is. While you are feeling that, allow yourself to breathe into the pose and let the breath lighten the pose for you, ignoring external distractions such as the noise you're hearing on the outside of this yoga studio, by focusing on listening to your breath, by intentionally making your inhale long and your exhale longer, regardless of how uncomfortable you are, you are starting to feel the pose. Notice that you become more aware of yourself than anything outside of yourself."

This was an "aha" moment for me. It felt like I learned how to shut off other people's judgments and views about me, focusing more on my feelings. As I kept on being mindful in my yoga practice, it broadened my understanding of why I started this fitness journey in the first place.

This enlightening experience highlighted the importance of understanding the "why" behind our actions. Initially, my weight loss journey began with the sting of rejection and a desire to alter others' perceptions of me. Through yoga, I realized that genuine transformation should be consciously rooted in self-love, not driven by the desire for external validation.

I also recognized that while a certain degree of external validation can be benign and motivating, it becomes problematic when it overshadows our concept of health and balance. Finding a balance, where self-worth is not exclusively tied to others' opinions but is anchored in our own positive self-image, is essential.

Furthermore, the journey underscored the irreplaceable value of guidance from seasoned professionals. Though we live in an age where information is readily available online, the personalized direction and support a knowledgeable coach or mentor can provide are invaluable. They offer a compass to navigate the complexities of transformations, ensuring decisions are grounded in a holistic understanding of health and well-being.

The adoption of this practice proved transformative in numerous ways. It taught me the resilience and strength of the human spirit—that with determination and the right mindset, our goals are within reach. More importantly, it highlighted the importance of seeking help and making informed choices for the right reasons. This comprehensive approach to health—considering both physical and mental dimensions—laid the foundation for sustainable well-being. It was a lesson in realizing that true contentment and fulfillment emanate from within, not from the metrics on a scale or the affirmation of others.

Chapter 8

Embracing the Balance

At the very heart of my transformative journey lay the transforming power of self- belief. This belief wasn't made up of fleeting thoughts, but a concrete conviction nurtured daily. It involved replacing years of self-doubt and criticism with positive affirmations through an ongoing dialogue with myself. This mental shift didn't take place overnight. It entailed a consistent effort to believe in my potential. Each day presented a new opportunity to celebrate small victories and learn from setbacks, constantly reminding myself of my ability to change.

Alongside self-belief, the path led me to develop sustainable health habits. My journey was one of trial and error as I experimented with various diets and exercises. The goal was to find helpful routines that were not just effective but also enjoyable and sustainable. Integrating healthy eating and physical activity became a natural and fulfilling part of my life, transforming them from chores to eagerly anticipated parts of my day.

Understanding and managing emotional eating was another profound aspect of my story. I delved deep into my inner self, confronting emotions and memories long suppressed with food. This process involved recognizing the triggers behind my terrible eating habits and adopting healthier coping mechanisms. It was about breaking the cycle of emotional eating by being mindful of why I was eating and choosing healthier responses like talking to a friend, going for a walk, or writing in a journal.

The journey was also immensely enriched by community and support. Friends, family, and online communities provided encouragement, understanding, and accountability. Sharing my experiences, both successes and struggles, systematically reinforced my commitment to my goals and served as a source of motivation and inspiration.

A particularly enlightening discovery was the true essence of body positivity. It's about more than just loving your body; it's about respecting and taking care of it healthfully. This realization led me to a balanced approach, where accepting my body and improving my health were not opposing objectives but complementary goals. Embracing body positivity meant recognizing that self-love and healthful living coexist. This approach involved understanding the importance of both mental and physical health and finding ways to nurture both. For instance, while I embraced my body's appearance, I also recognized the need for regular exercise, balanced nutrition, and mental well-being. This holistic view of body positivity shifted my perspective from merely accepting to actively nurturing my body, leading to an overall improvement in my health and well-being.

Finally, the role of habit tracking in sustaining my transformation was a key element. Using various tools to keep a comprehensive record of my eating habits, exercise routines, and emotional states played a significant role in my journey. This tracking provided concrete data about my progress, helping me make informed adjustments. It also served as a motivational tool, constantly reminding me of how far I had come and reinforcing my commitment to my health goals.

As I share these insights, I hope to inspire those embarking on their individual journeys toward a balanced and fulfilling life.

Conclusion

A Journey to Holistic Well-Being

Reflecting on my unique journey, as narrated in "How I Lost 155 Pounds in 10 Months," I realize it encompassed much more than weight loss. This path was a profound learning experience about loving and respecting my body, nurturing my mental health, and embracing a balanced life.

My childhood was filled with struggles of ridicule and isolation. Yet, it was the warmth of new friendships, like when Mark joined me for lunch one day, seeing past my size and connecting with me on a deeper level, that ignited my transformation. These experiences taught me resilience and growth.

The gym, which I initially saw as intimidating, became a much-needed sanctuary of self-improvement. I still remember my first successful treadmill run; it was more than just exercise; it was overcoming a mental barrier.

Food, once a source of comfort during stressful times, evolved into a balanced part of my life. Learning to see food as nourishing fuel rather than an emotional crutch was a critical part of my transformation. I recall the first time I chose a salad over fast food during a hectic workday – a small victory, but a significant step in my journey.

True body positivity emerged as a central lesson. It meant respecting my body, which went beyond mere acceptance of its shape. I recall the day I confidently chose to wear my swimming trunk at the beach, embracing my body with pride. This shift was about making healthful choices, not just to conform to societal pressures but for my overall well-being.

Habit tracking became a crucial tool, gradually transforming small steps into significant milestones. The satisfaction of marking a full month of consistent gym attendance was a testament to this.

The support from friends, family, and the online community was invaluable. Their encouragement and empathy, like the time a friend joined me for a morning jog despite the rain, were pillars of my journey.

As I move forward, I carry these lessons with me, applying them to all aspects of my life. This journey has evolved into a lifelong commitment to a balanced, healthy, and fulfilling existence, marked by continuous learning and growth.

For those who see a reflection of their struggles in this story, let it be a source of hope. Change is achievable, and transformation is possible. This journey has taught me the importance of balance, self-belief, perseverance, and embracing a balanced life.

Thank you for being part of this journey. I hope my story inspires you to embark on your own transformative path of health, self-discovery, and fulfillment.

With a heart full of gratitude and renewed hope, —Brian.

Epilogue

BEYOND THE SCALE - A LIFE TRANSFORMED

As I reflect on the incredible journey narrated in "How I Lost 155 Pounds in 10 Months," I find myself in a remarkably different place from where I started. Gone are the days of the monotonous 9-5 job that once defined my existence. Now, at a steady weight of 165 pounds and standing 5ft 10in tall, my life has taken a turn I could have never foreseen.

During my transformation journey, I crossed paths with Dave, who would become not just my partner but also a pillar of strength and support. He entered my life as I grappled with the mental and emotional challenges that accompanied my physical transformation. Witnessing my struggles with wanting to lose more weight, he provided me with a perspective that was grounded in compassion and understanding.

Together, we embarked on a venture that has become our shared passion and purpose. We established a Yoga studio and wellness center in my hometown, a venture born out of our mutual love for health and well-being. This center has become a haven for many seeking solace and a path to better health, offering a range of services that cater to physical fitness, mental clarity, and emotional well-being.

The onset of the COVID-19 pandemic brought unforeseen challenges, but it also opened doors to new possibilities. Recognizing the need for connection and well-being in a time of isolation and uncertainty, Dave and I launched an online yoga platform. Initially, it was our way of extending support to those confined at home, offering them an easy means to maintain their physical health and find mental peace amidst the turmoil. What started as a small initiative to keep people engaged and healthy during lockdowns blossomed into a thriving online community.

Our online platform has become more than just a virtual space for yoga; it's a community where people from all walks of life come together to share their journeys, triumphs, and struggles. It's a place where isolation is combated with connection, where physical distance is bridged by digital togetherness. The growth of this platform has been a heartwarming reminder of the universal need for community and the power of yoga to unite.

Back in our physical studio, the growth has been equally inspiring. Every new member who walks through our doors brings their unique story, adding to the rich tapestry of our community. From beginners taking their first steps in yoga to seasoned practitioners deepening their practice, each individual contributes to the vibrant energy of our space.

Reflecting on this journey, I am struck by how much my life has changed. My pursuit of weight loss has, in fact, evolved into a broader quest for holistic health and community building. The lessons I've learned extend far beyond the realms of diet and exercise. They are about the power of resilience, the importance of mental and emotional health, and the joy of sharing wellness with others.

Before And After Pictures

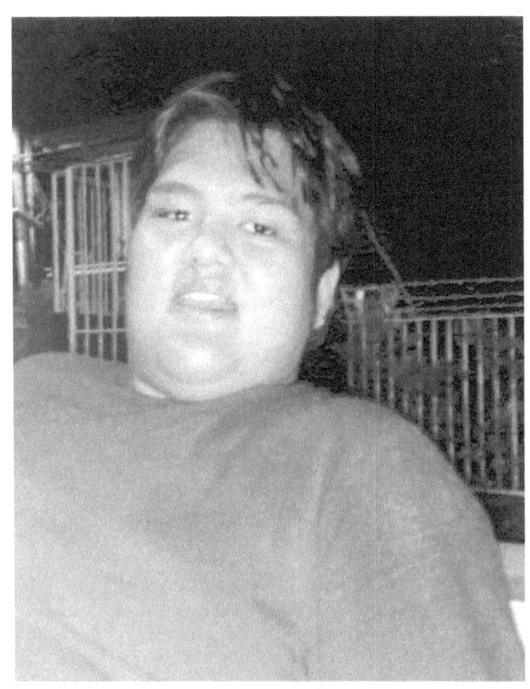

Brian - Before

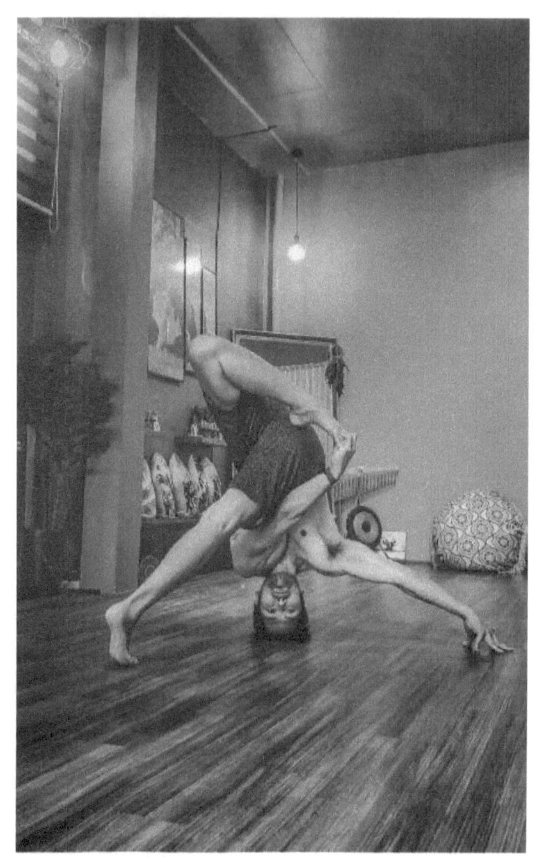

Brian Tranforming His Body

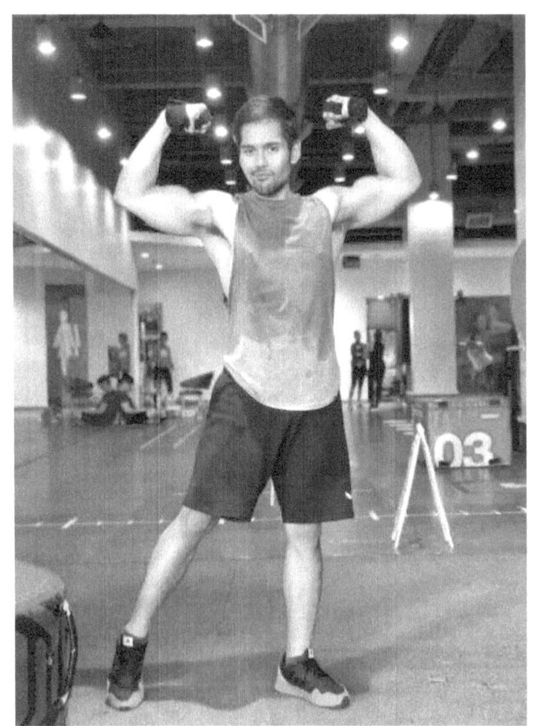

Brian After

Joining Hands, Moving Forward

I extend an invitation to you to join our community. This community celebrates every step toward a healthier self, acknowledging the highs and lows and offering mutual support through each of our unique journeys. Here, you'll find a group of individuals committed to making positive life changes. In our community, we share experiences, learn from one another, and grow together. It's a space not just about weight loss or fitness goals; it's about nurturing our overall well-being, discovering joy in our journey, and cultivating self-love.

My journey has taught me that transformation transcends physical change. It's about finding balance, understanding our motivations, and forging robust connections with those who uplift and inspire us.

I invite you to join us on this path of health, happiness, and holistic well-being. Together, let's share our stories, celebrate our achievements, and provide support in challenging times. United, we can accomplish more than we ever thought possible!

Join us on Instagram: instagram.com/braveyoga.ph

Join us on Facebook: facebook.com/braveyogaph

Follow me on Instagram: instagram.com/brine4u

Facebook Community Group Page: braveyogacommunity

BRAVEYOGA.PH

Bonus Content

Unlocking Your Body's Energy Codes: Your Guide to Calculating BMR and TDEE

Introduction: Welcome to a key part of your wellness journey! Understanding your body's energy requirements is crucial in your path to health and fitness. In this section, we'll explore how to calculate your Basal Metabolic Rate (BMR) and Total Daily Energy Expenditure (TDEE), essential tools for tailoring your weight loss plan.

Understanding Your Basal Metabolic Rate (BMR): Your BMR is the number of calories your body needs to perform basic life-sustaining functions. This includes breathing, circulation, cell production, nutrient processing, and temperature regulation.

Factors Influencing Your BMR:

- **Age:** BMR decreases with age.

- **Gender:** Men typically have a higher BMR than women.

- **Weight and Height:** More weight and height generally mean a higher BMR.

- **Muscle Mass:** Muscle burns more calories at rest than fat.

The BMR Formula calculates the number of calories your body needs to perform basic life-sustaining functions while at rest. There are several formulas to calculate BMR, but one of the most commonly used is the Harris-Benedict Equation. It considers your age, sex, weight, and height to estimate your BMR. The formulas are as follows:

For Men: BMR = 88.362 + (13.397 x weight in kg) + (4.799 x height in cm) - (5.677 x age in years)

For Women: BMR = 447.593 + (9.247 x weight in kg) + (3.098 x height in cm) - (4.330 x age in years)

This equation provides an estimate of how many calories you would burn per day if you were at rest all day. It's important to note that this is a basic estimation and actual calorie needs can vary based on other factors like muscle mass, physical activity, and overall health.

Calculating Your Total Daily Energy Expenditure (TDEE): TDEE is the total number of calories you burn in a day when exercise is taken into account. It's your BMR plus the energy expended through physical activity.

Activity Levels and TDEE:

- **Sedentary** (little to no exercise): BMR x 1.2

- **Lightly Active** (light exercise 1-3 days/week): BMR x 1.375

- **Moderately Active** (moderate exercise 3-5 days/week): BMR x 1.55

- **Very Active** (hard exercise 6-7 days a week): BMR x 1.725

Understanding your Basal Metabolic Rate (BMR) and Total Daily Energy Expenditure (TDEE) is important for managing weight because:

1. **Knowing Your Body's Calorie Needs:** BMR tells you the minimum calories your body needs to function at rest. This helps you understand how many calories you need just to maintain your basic bodily functions.

2. **Tailoring Your Diet and Exercise:** TDEE includes calories burned through daily activities and exercise. Knowing this helps you plan your diet and exercise according to whether you want to lose, gain, or maintain weight.

3. **Creating a Caloric Deficit or Surplus:**

   - **For Losing Weight:** You need to eat fewer calories than your TDEE. This means you're using more energy than you're consuming, leading to weight loss.

   - **For Gaining Weight:** You need to eat more calories than your TDEE. This surplus helps in weight gain, especially if you're trying to build muscle.

4. **Adapting as You Go:** As you lose or gain weight, your calorie needs change. Knowing your BMR and TDEE helps you adjust your diet and exercise plans over time.

Putting It Into Practice: Now that you know your BMR and TDEE, use these numbers to plan your diet and exercise regimen. Remember, to lose weight, you'll need to create a calorie deficit.

Free Webinar

Join Our Free Webinar! For more insights and personalized guidance, join our free webinar at http://bit.ly/braveyoga. Dive deeper into understanding your body's needs and how to effectively manage your wellness journey. See you there!